The Kitchen Beautician: Natural Hair Care Recipes for Beautiful Healthy Hair

By Dezarae Henderson

This book is dedicated to all women of the world exploring, learning, embracing and loving their natural hair texture. There is something inside of this book for everyone.

I would like to thank all of my friends and family for supporting me. TJ, thank you for understanding how important my Sunday hair days are and staying out of the kitchen! ☺ I love you.

You inspire me each and every day. This one is for you.

III

Table of Contents

1. Scrumptious Shampoos   Page 4
2. Delectable Dry Shampoos   Page 14
3. Captivating Conditioners   Page 17
4. Tasty Treatments and Rinses   Page 43
5. Charming Colors   Page 57
6. Succulent Styling Products   Page 65
7. Helpful Hints   Page 77

Scrumptious Shampoos

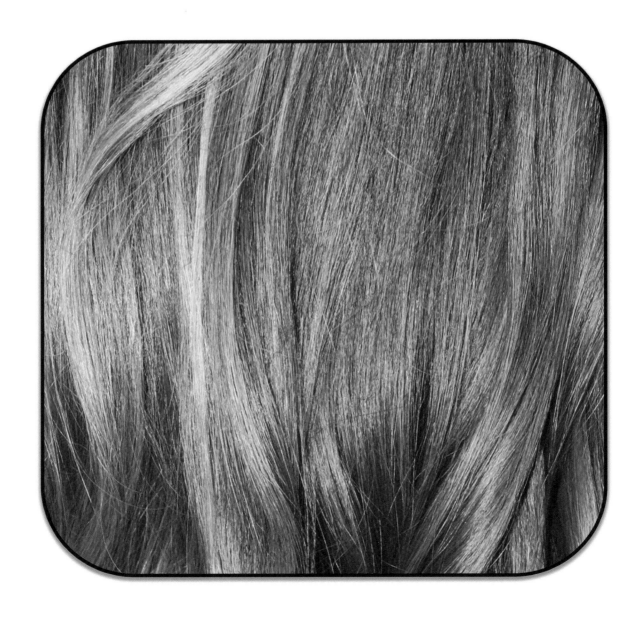

A Drizzle of Olive Oil Shampoo

For Dry Hair

Ingredients:

¼ cup liquid castile soap

¼ tsp. olive oil

¼ cup aloe vera gel

1 tsp. glycerine

Combine ingredients into a medium sized bowl. Mix thoroughly. Pour mixture into an empty shampoo bottle and shake vigorously. Due to the shampoo not including preservatives, ingredients may separate between uses. Shake the bottle prior to each use.

𝒫airs well with: Piña Colada Conditioner (see recipe page 22)

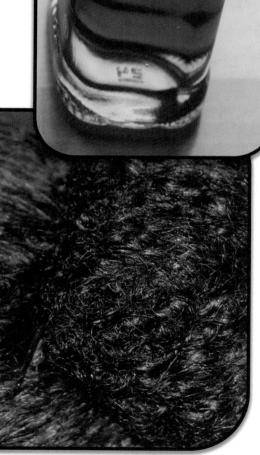

Tea Cakes Shampoo

Organic Shampoo

Ingredients:

2 oz. water

1 organic rosemary tea bag

8 oz. organic liquid castile soap

1 tbsp. organic lemon juice

1 tbsp. baking soda

1/4 tsp. grapefruit seed extract

Heat water to boiling in a small saucepan. Once boiling, remove the saucepan from heat. Steep tea bag in the water for 10 minutes. Remove the tea bag from the water and discard. Add soap, lemon juice, baking soda and grapefruit seed extract to the water. Heat the mixture over low heat, while stirring constantly, until the mixture is fully combined. Remove mixture from the heat and leave it to cool for 30 minutes. Pour the organic shampoo into a clean bottle. Be sure to shake prior to each use.

Pairs well with: AvoCoco Guacamole Conditioner (see page 26)

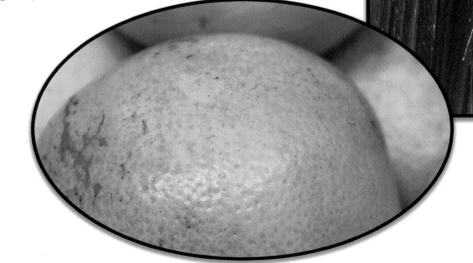

Essentially Normal Shampoo

For Normal Hair

Ingredients:

½ cup distilled water

½ cup liquid castile soap

1 tsp. olive oil

1 tsp. coconut oil

10 drops essential oil (optional)

Combine distilled water and castile soap. Mix well until both ingredients are uniform. Add in the coconut and olive oil. Pour concoction into an empty bottle and shake vigorously. Add your favorite essential oil for scent.

*P*airs well with: Brilliant Brewed Conditioner (see page 27)

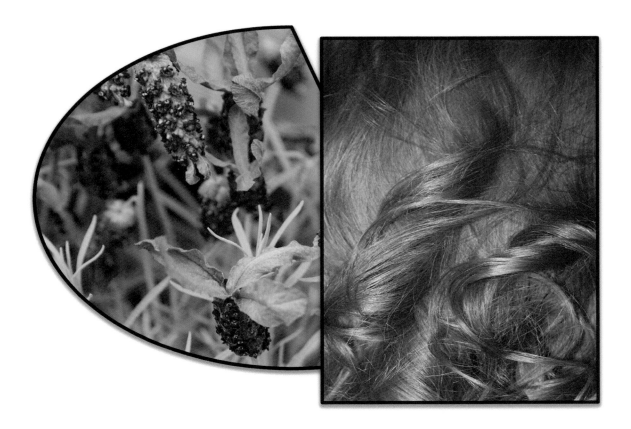

Peppermint Ribbons Shampoo

Moisturizing Shampoo

Ingredients:

1/3 cup distilled water

2/3 cup liquid castile soap

1 tsp. sea salt

3 tsp. jojoba oil

1 tsp. coconut oil

10 drops peppermint essential oil

Combine distilled water and castile soap. Mix well until ingredients are uniform. Add in sea salt and stir until completely dissolved. Stir in jojoba and coconut oil and transfer contents into an empty shampoo bottle. Drop in peppermint oil for scalp stimulation and shake contents vigorously. Be sure to shake the shampoo before each use for maximum benefits.

*P*airs well with: Shea Anything Conditioner (see page 23)

Nettle the Itch Away Shampoo

Itch-Relief Natural Shampoo

Ingredients:

8 oz. water

3 oz. castile soap

1 tsp. stinging nettles

1 tsp. lavender

Bring water to a boil. Once boiling, add in stinging nettles and lavender. For best results, cover the pot and let the concoction simmer for at least 20 minutes. Strain the mixture with a colander to remove the herbs and let the liquid cool to room temperature.   Transfer contents into an empty shampoo bottle and add castile soap. Shake contents vigorously until mixture is uniform.

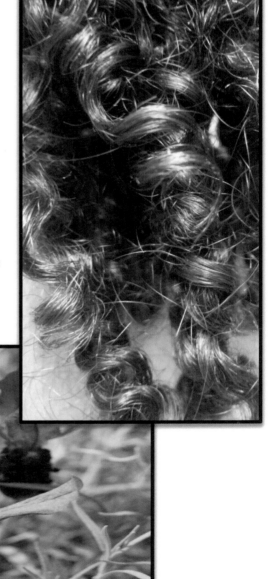

*P*airs well with: Apple of Your Eye Conditioner (see page 19)

Mint Julipoo Shampoo

Natural Shampoo for Oily Hair

Ingredients:

2 cups distilled water

2 tbsp. peppermint leaves

2 tbsp. spearmint leaves

1 tbsp. dried sage

½ cup liquid castile soap

5 drops lavender essential oil

Bring water to a boil. Add peppermint, spearmint and sage to the pot. Cover the pot and let the concoction steep for at least 15 minutes to allow for the herbs to release its flavors.   Strain the mixture using a colander and discard the herbs. Mix in the liquid castile soap and transfer concoction to an empty shampoo bottle. Add lavender oil to the mixture and shake vigorously to ensure ingredients are properly mixed.

*P*airs well with: Bananas Foster conditioner (see page 18)

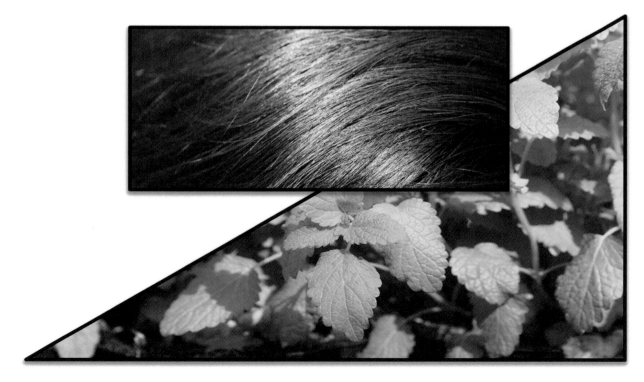

Clean Squeaky Clean Without Soap!

Soap-less Shampoo

Ingredients:

¼ cup baking soda

8-10 oz. water, depending on hair length

Combine the baking soda with water. Create a paste-like consistency by adding more water or more baking soda depending on hair length. Generously apply mixture to hair from scalp to the end of the hair strands. The baking soda granules will exfoliate hair strands to leave hair squeaky clean and soft to the touch.

*Note- Soap-less shampoo does not produce lather but it still cleans your hair quite well.

𝒫airs well with: Oats and Avocado Milkshake Hair Mask (see page 20)

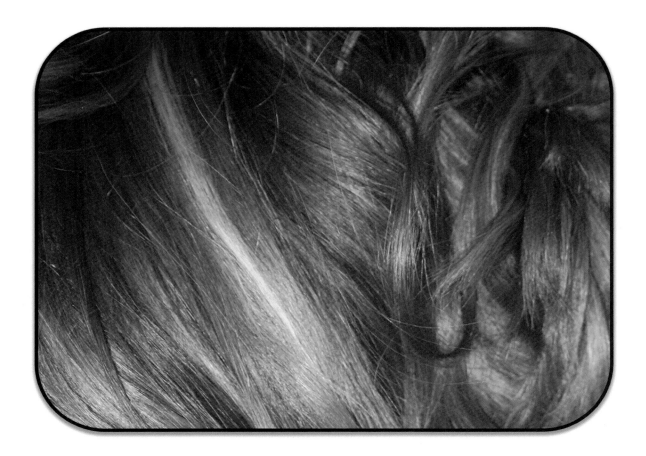

Honey, I'm Home Shampoo

Honey and Aloe Shampoo

Ingredients:

¼ cup aloe vera gel

2 tbsp. honey

2 tbsp. apple cider vinegar

Mix ingredients and apply to hair generously. Leave on for 3-5 minutes and rinse thoroughly. Follow up with a moisturizing conditioner.

Pairs well with: Eggs Sunnyside Up Conditioner (see page 21)

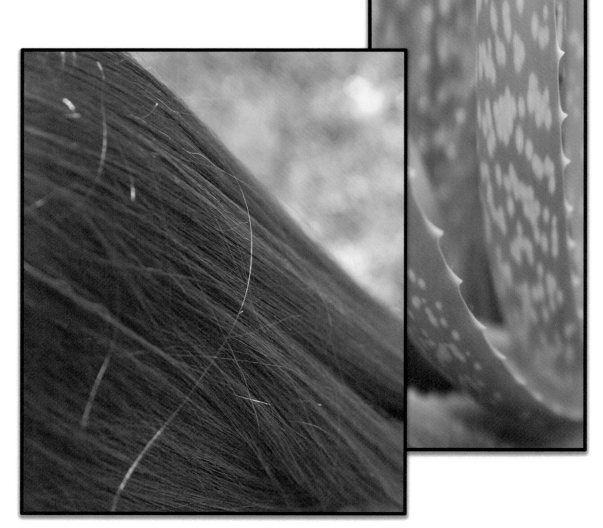

All Together Now Shampoo and Conditioner

All in one shampoo/conditioner

Ingredients:

1 ripe Avocado

2 tbsp. baking soda

4 tbsp. distilled Water

Mash the avocado into a paste then add the baking soda and water until you have a nice even paste (about the same consistency as a regular shampoo/conditioner). Rinse your hair with warm water to open the hair cuticles, which will aid in cleansing the hair. Apply the shampoo/conditioner throughout your hair starting at the roots and working your way to the ends. Let it sit for 5 minutes and rinse it out with lukewarm water, slowly transitioning the water to a cool. This will close the cuticles again for a shinier and smoother look and will leave your hair silky smooth.

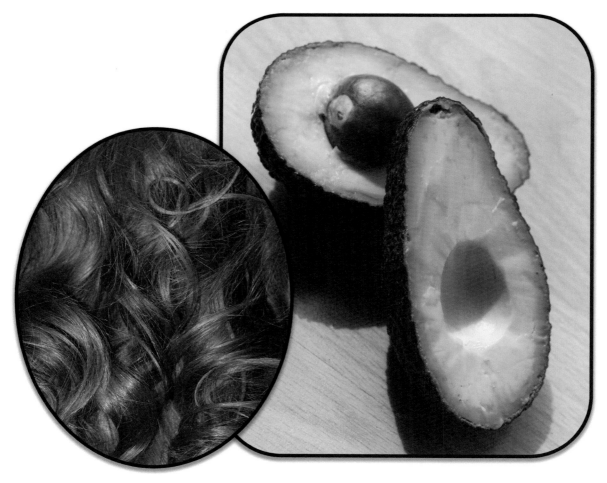

Delectable Dry Shampoos

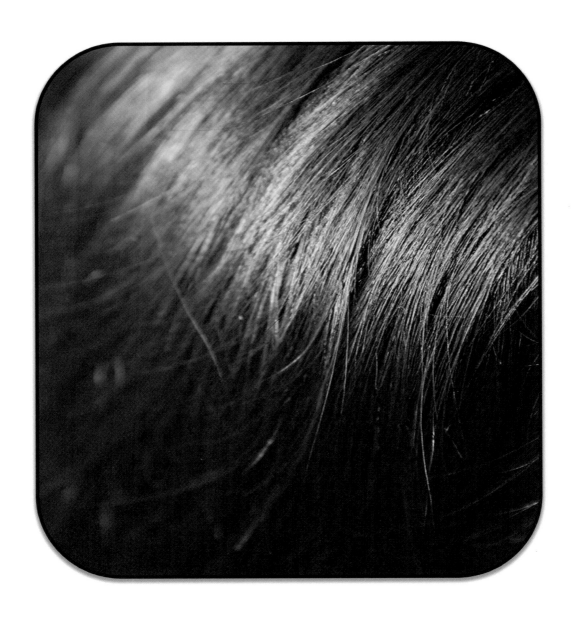

Corn-on-the Cob Dry Shampoo

Natural Cornstarch Dry Shampoo

Cornstarch

Add a little bit of cornstarch to your roots. Then, blend it through your hair. Finally, brush the cornstarch out of your hair. The cornstarch soaks up the oil and dirt and leaves your hair fresh and clean.

Salty Sea Dry Shampoo

Salt and Cornmeal Dry Shampoo

1 tsp. salt

½ cup cornmeal

Mix salt and cornmeal. Pour mixture into a salt or pepper shaker. Shake the mixture on your hair and brush it out. As you brush, oil and dirt are instantly removed.

Mac n' Cheesecloth Dry Shampoo

Cheesecloth Dry Shampoo

Cheesecloth

No ingredients needed! Simply wrap the cheesecloth around a wide natural bristle brush and then brush your hair. The cheesecloth will remove any dirt and oil from your hair.

Just Claying Around Dry Shampoo

Clarifying Dry Clay Shampoo

Powdered clay

Powdered milk

Use any dry clay such as agar agar, white or green clay and add in an even amount of powdered milk depending on the length of your hair. Work the mixture into your roots and then brush out. Clay will naturally remove the oil from your hair so the powdered milk is important for adding back moisture.

Clean as a Baby's Bottom Dry Shampoo

Baby powder Dry Shampoo

Baby Powder

Baking Soda

This is one of the most common methods of making a dry shampoo. Mix even amounts of baby powder and baking soda depending on the length of your hair. Rub the mixture into the roots of your hair and brush hair from root to tips to distribute the shampoo down the hair strands. Baking soda will provide instant cleanse and baby powder will leave a pleasant scent.

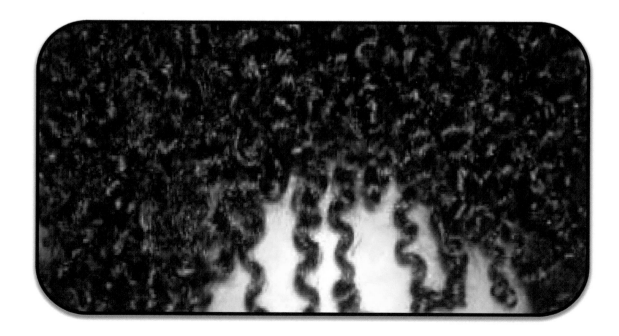

Captivating Conditioners

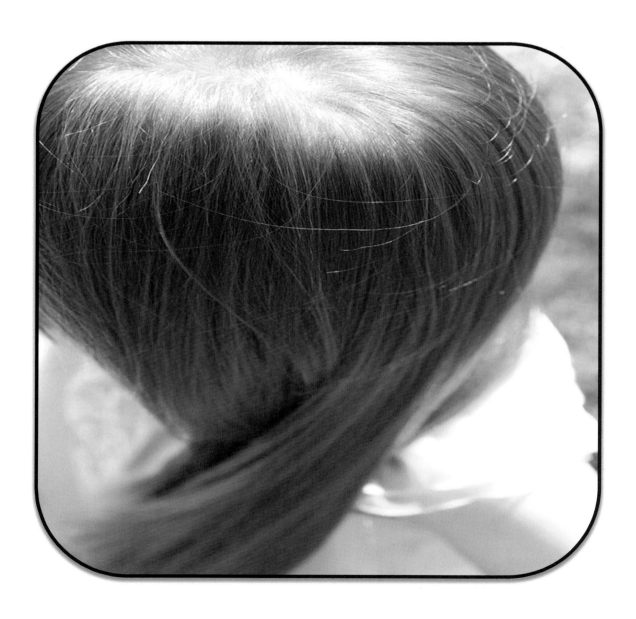

Bananas Foster Conditioner

For Manageability

Ingredients:

1 large overripe banana or 7 oz. banana baby food

4 tbsp. extra virgin olive oil

2 tbsp. pure vegetable glycerin

2 tbsp. honey

Place the ingredients in a blender and blend the ingredients thoroughly, ensuring there are no remaining lumps. (Depending on the quality of your blender, you may need to pour the mixture through a sieve. Using banana baby food omits any lumps, but the conditioner may not be as effective.) Apply to hair and let sit for 30-45 minutes under a shower cap. Rinse thoroughly and style as usual.

*P*airs well with: Mint Julipoo Shampoo (see page 10)

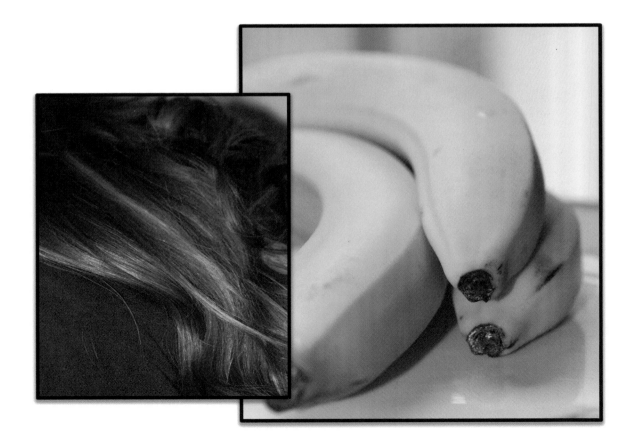

Apple of Your Eye Conditioner

Detangling Conditioner

Ingredients:

1 overripe avocado, sliced

¼ cup extra virgin olive oil

½ cup unrefined shea butter

2-3 tbsp. apple cider vinegar

Place the sliced avocado, shea butter, olive oil and apple cider vinegar in a blender. Blend the ingredients thoroughly and add more olive oil, if necessary, until the mixture reaches your desired consistency. Apply to hair and let sit for 30-45 minutes under a shower cap. Rinse thoroughly and style as usual.

*P*airs well with: Nettle the Itch Away Shampoo (see page 9)

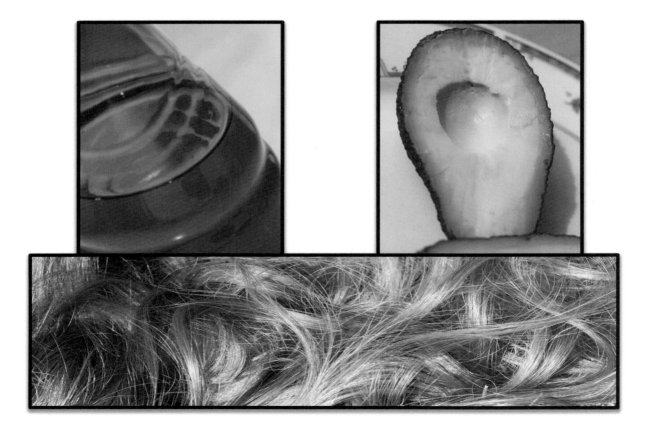

Oats and Avocado Milkshake Hair Mask

Mask for Dry and/or Curly Hair Types

Ingredients:

1 overripe avocado

¼ cup rolled or steel-cut oats

1 cup milk (for extra moisture, use goat's milk)

1/8-1/4 cup olive oil, depending on hair condition.

Mash the avocado into a paste then add the oatmeal. Consistency should be thick at this point. Stir in milk and olive oil and blend until mixture is smooth. (Add additional olive oil for dry or damaged hair.) Apply generously to clean damp hair and let sit for 30 minutes. Rinse with lukewarm water and transition the temperature to cool in order to seal the cuticles.

*P*airs well with: Squeaky Clean Without Soap! (see page 11)

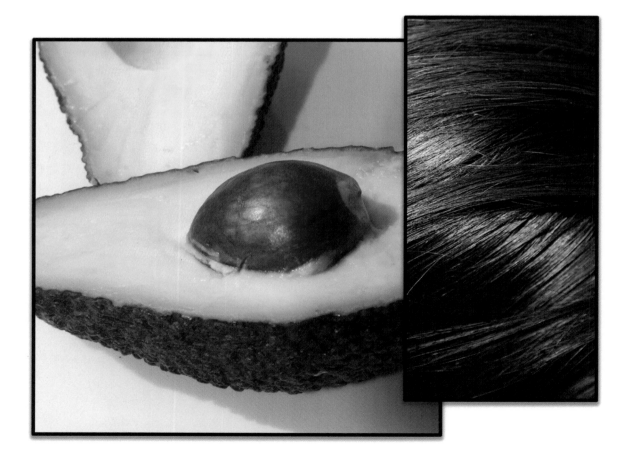

Eggs Sunny Side Up Conditioner

Deep Protein Conditioner

Ingredients:

4 tbsp. mayonnaise

1 egg

1 tbsp. extra virgin olive oil

1 tbsp. extra virgin coconut oil

3 tbsp. organic honey

4 drops peppermint essential oil

4 drops rosemary essential oil

Combine all ingredients in a mixing bowl and mix well. Cover hair root to tip with the mixture and cover with a plastic cap for extra conditioning. Leave it on for at least an hour and rinse out with very cool water to seal cuticles and prevent the egg from cooking in your hair.

*P*airs well with: Honey, I'm Home Shampoo (see page 12)

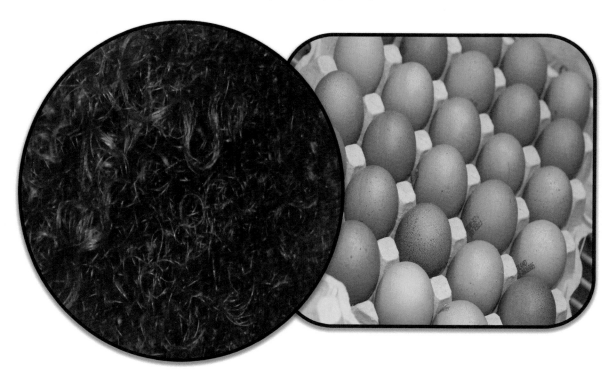

Piña Colada Conditioner

Moisturizing Deep Penetrating Conditioner

Ingredients:

1 2.5 oz. jar banana baby food

¼ cup coconut cream or milk (Cream provides more moisture)

1 tbsp. honey

1 tbsp. coconut or avocado oil

10 drops essential oil (optional)

Combine all ingredients in a bowl until smooth. Add additional coconut cream, honey or oil to make conditioner more moisturizing, if desired. This conditioner can be scented with 10 drops of the essential oil of your choice. Apply generously to the hair from root to tip with the mixture and cover with a plastic cap and a warm towel. Leave the conditioner on for at least 30 minutes then rinse with cool water.

Pairs well with: A Drizzle of Olive Oil Shampoo (see page 5)

Shea Anything Conditioner

Shea Butter and Honey Conditioner

Ingredients:

2 eggs

2 tbsp. shea butter

2 tbsp. honey

½ banana

1 tbsp. aloe vera

Combine all the ingredients in a blender and blend until smooth. Massage mixture into hair and cover with a shower cap or warm towel for at least 10 minutes. Be cautious when using heat as the egg may cook while in the hair.

*P*airs well with:
Peppermint Ribbons Shampoo (see page 8)

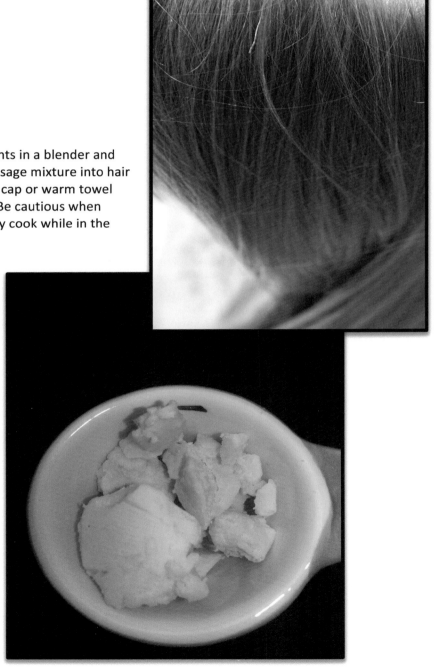

Quick Protein On-the-Go

Simple Protein Treatment

Ingredients:

8 oz. mayonnaise

1/2 avocado

Peel avocado and remove pit. Mix all ingredients in a medium-sized bowl until smooth in texture. Smooth into hair being careful to work it to the ends. Use shower cap or plastic wrap to seal body heat in. Leave on hair for 20 minutes. For deeper conditioning, wrap a hot, damp towel around your head over the plastic, or use a hair dryer set to a low to medium heat setting.

*P*airs well with: Nettle the Itch Away Shampoo (see page 9)

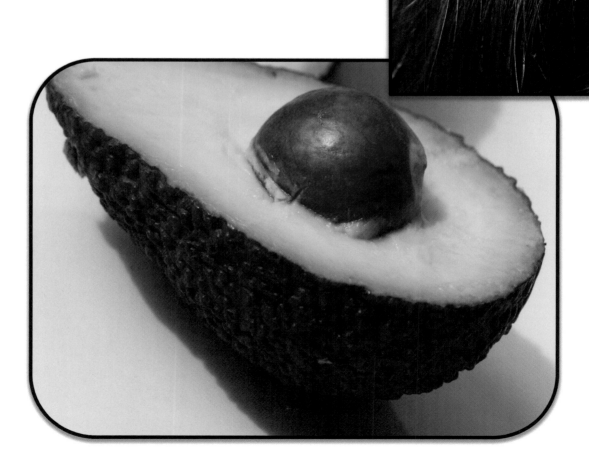

AvoCoco Guacamole Conditioner

Ingredients:

1 avocado

Organic coconut milk

Peel the avocado and remove the pit. Mash avocado and slowly add coconut milk until mixture is smooth and the desired consistency. Work through hair to ends. Rinse after 15 minutes and shampoo.

Pairs well with: Tea Cakes Shampoo (see page 6)

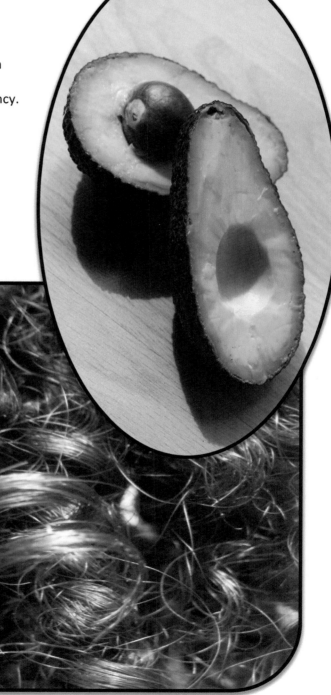

Brilliant Brewed Conditioner

Beer Conditioner

Ingredients:

1 cup warm beer

1 tsp. jojoba oil

Mix all ingredients until smooth. Apply to hair and massage through. Rinse well with cold water. Beer provides instant shine to hair.

*P*airs well with: Honey, I'm Home Shampoo (see page 12)

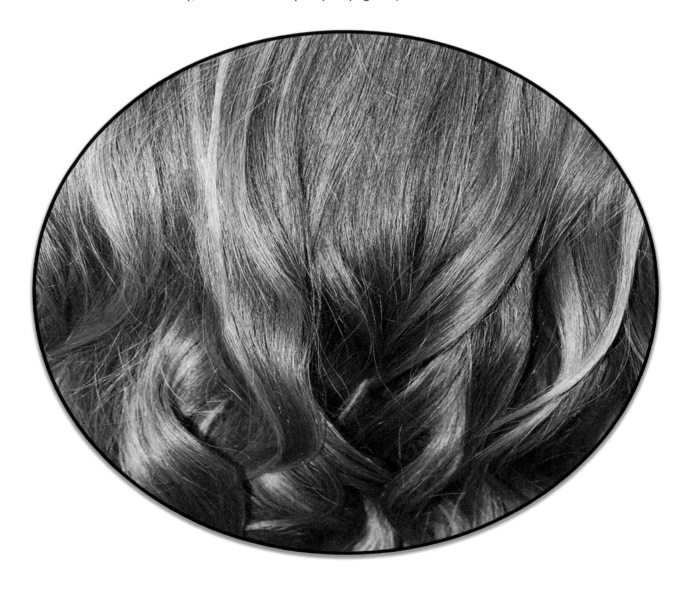

Plucky Persimmon Conditioner

Persimmon and Rosemary Conditioner

Ingredients:

1 ripe persimmon

1 sprig rosemary

1/4 cup almond oil

1/2 cup honey

5-10 drops peppermint essential oil

Chop up the persimmon into small pieces and pulse it in the food processor to make it even finer. Add rosemary, almond oil, honey and peppermint oil. Continue to blend in the processor until it is smooth and creamy in texture.   Apply mixture to hair and rinse with cool water.

*P*airs well with: Mint Julipoo Shampoo (see page 10)

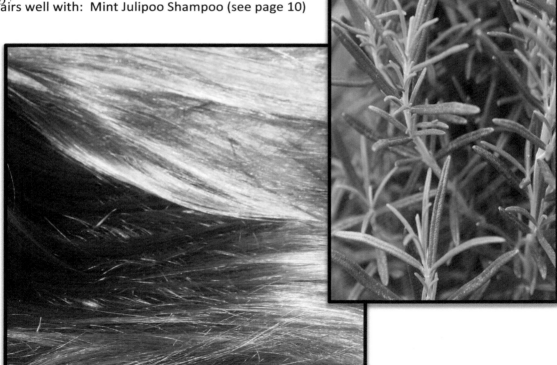

Eggs Benedict Conditioner

Avocado & Egg Conditioner

Ingredients:

1 avocado

2 egg yolks

Peel the avocado and mash it into a paste. Place 1 cup of the avocado paste inside a bowl then add the yolk of two eggs. Beat the mixture and apply to hair. Leave on for 30 minutes then rinse out.

𝒫airs well with: Peppermint Ribbons Shampoo (see page 8)

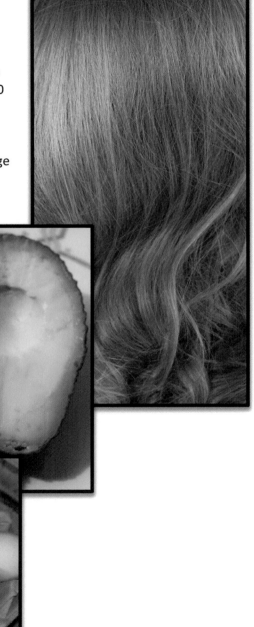

Coconut Grove Conditioner

Tropical Conditioner

Ingredients:

1 avocado

Coconut milk

Peel and smash the avocado into a paste. Place into a bowl and add coconut milk. Mix together until smooth and keep the texture thick. Comb thru hair and leave it on for 10-15 minutes. Rinse out with cool water.

*P*airs well with: Essentially Normal Shampoo (see page 7)

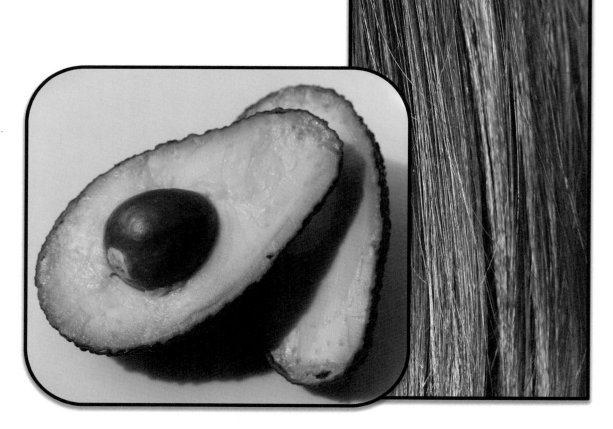

Lemon Meringue Conditioner

Sunflower Hair Conditioner

Ingredients:

1 cup sunflower oil

1 cup wheat germ oil

1 tsp. lemon juice

Add sunflower oil and wheat germ oil in a blender and blend together until well combined. Heat the mixture a little in the microwave for a few seconds. Apply onto hair for a few minutes then wash it out with lukewarm water. Add the lemon juice to the lukewarm water during the final rinse.

*P*airs well with: Tea Cakes Shampoo (see page 6)

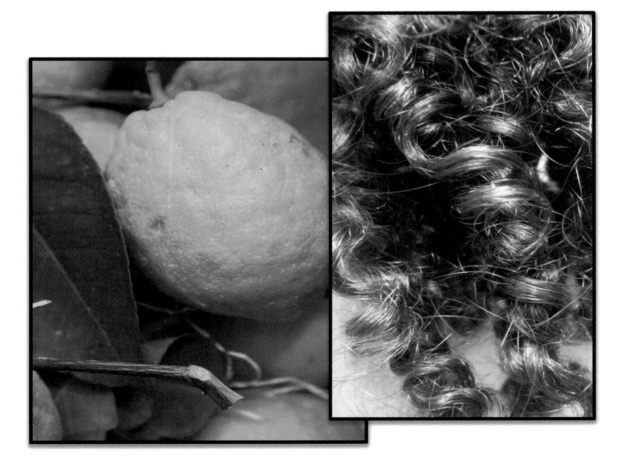

Hydrating Henna Conditioner

For Dry Hair

Ingredients:

3.5 oz. powdered henna

1 tbsp. olive oil

Milk

Place henna in a bowl and add olive oil. Add warm milk until mixture is thick and well combined. Apply to the hair for 20 minutes. Rinse out with lukewarm water.

Pairs well with: Tea Cakes Shampoo (see page 6)

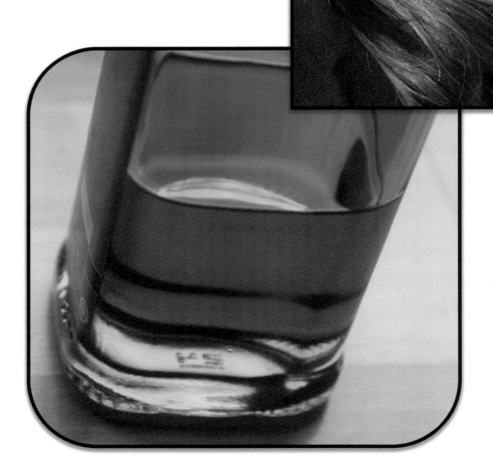

Curds and Whey Conditioner

For Oily Hair

Ingredients:

3.5 oz. powdered henna

2 tbsp. curd

Pinch of sugar

Water

Place henna in a bowl and add curd and sugar. Add water until mixture is thick and well combined. Apply to the hair for 20 minutes. Rinse out with lukewarm water.

Pairs well with: Honey, I'm Home Shampoo (see page 12)

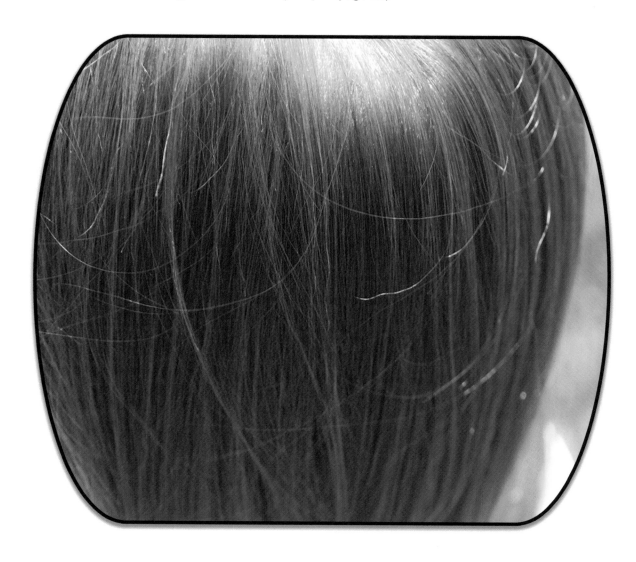

I'll Have The Works Conditioner

Ingredients:

1 avocado, peeled and mashed

1 small, ripe banana

½ cup coconut milk

½ cup flat beer

1 tsp. olive oil

2 egg yolks

1 tbsp. lemon juice

1 tbsp. apple cider vinegar

2 drops essential oil (optional)

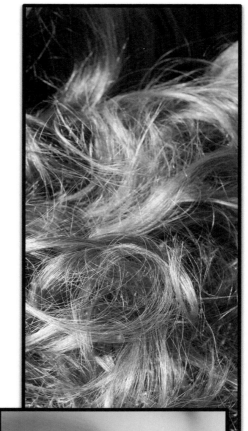

Mash all ingredients together until smooth and the consistency of a paste. Adjust consistency of mixture by adding more coconut milk, if necessary. Part your hair into small sections and apply the conditioner from hair roots to ends. Put shower cap on and cover with a towel to seal in treatment. Leave in for 20-30 minutes. Rinse out the mixture with cool water. Store leftovers in the refrigerator for future use.

Pairs well with: Nettle the Itch Away Shampoo
(see page 9)

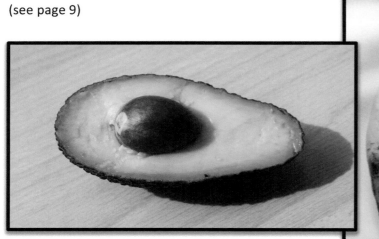

Little White Lies Conditioner

Degreasing Conditioner for Oily Hair

Ingredients:

1 egg white

½ cup distilled water

Warm up the distilled water until it is comfortably warm. Separate the egg white and gently whisk it while adding the warm water until you get a nice and smooth mixture. Apply it through your hair starting at your roots and slowly work your way to the ends. Leave it in for 5 minutes then rinse with lukewarm water. Follow up with a leave-in conditioner.

One of the best ingredients in a natural hair conditioner recipe is simple egg white. Egg whites absorb excess oil from your hair and make it look smooth and clean

Pairs well with: Allow for Vera Soft Hair Leave-In Conditioner (see page 39)

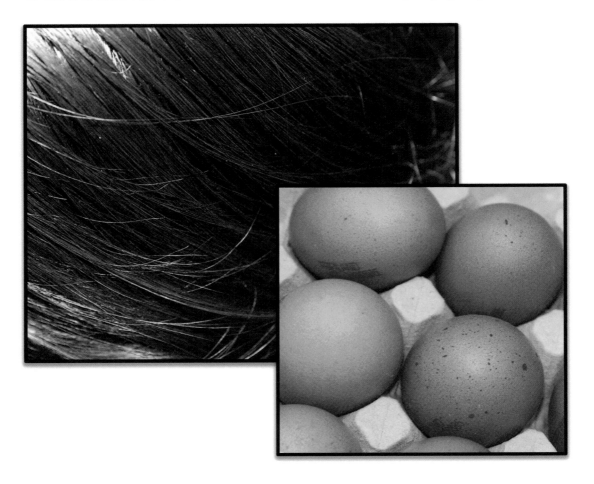

Frozen Yogurt Conditioner

Mayo, Egg Whites & Yogurt Conditioner

Ingredients:

8 tbsp. plain yogurt

8 tbsp. mayonnaise

1 egg white

Separate the egg white and gently whisk it then blend it with the yogurt and mayonnaise. Work it evenly through your hair starting at your roots and work your way to the ends, which should get a bit of extra attention. Put on a plastic shower cap or wrap your head in plastic wrap and let it sit for 30 minutes.   Rinse with lukewarm water.

*P*airs well with: Mint Julipoo Shampoo (see page 10)

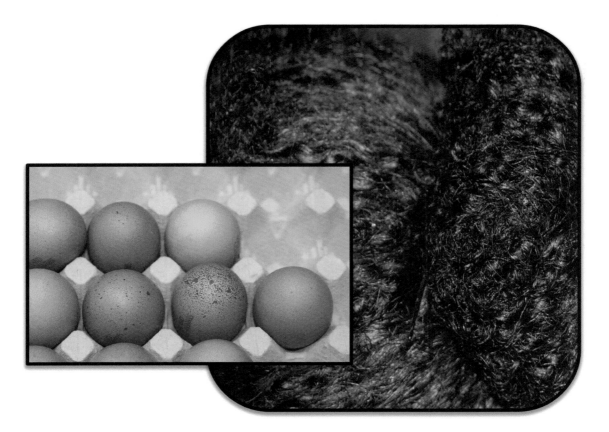

Comely Coconut Cream Conditioner

Conditioner for Dry & Frizzy Hair

Ingredients:

1 ripe avocado

1 cup coconut milk

2 tbsp. coconut oil

Cut the avocado, take out the pit and scoop out the fleshy meat and mash this into a nice paste. Add coconut milk and oil and mix until you get an evenly blended mixture. Work it into your hair and let it sit for 15 minutes. Rinse out with lukewarm water.

Pairs well with: Honey, I'm Home Shampoo (see page 12)

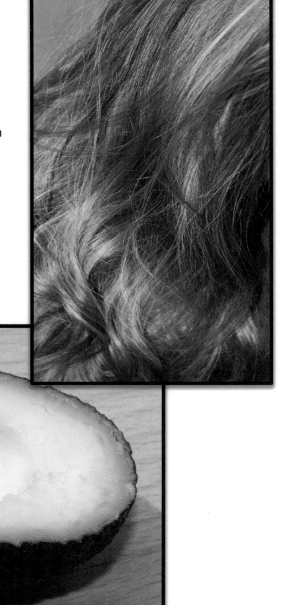

Shea's Hair Splitting Conditioner

Conditioner for Split Ends

Ingredients:

1 cup shea butter

5 tbsp. extra virgin olive oil

½ tsp. vitamin E oil

10 drops essential oil (optional)

Slowly warm up the shea butter until it melts. Remove from heat and stir in the olive oil. Let the mixture cool down for about 30 minutes, but don't let it set entirely. Mix in the vitamin E and essential oil while gently whisking it. Whisk until you get a conditioner-like consistency. Leftovers should be stored in an airtight container.

Pairs well with: Tea Cakes Shampoo (see page 6)

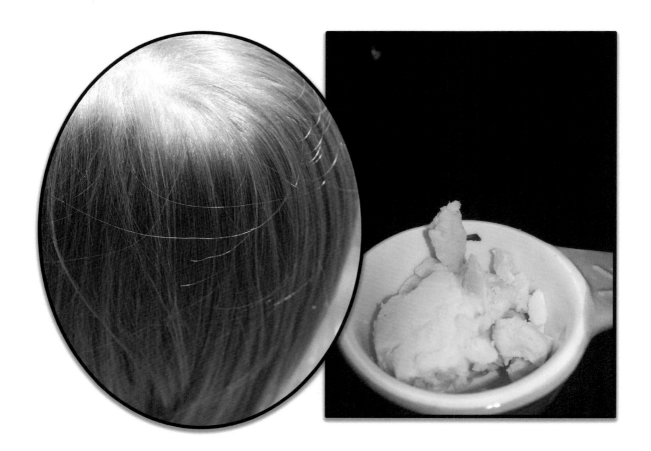

Allow for Vera Soft Hair Leave-In Conditioner

Aloe Vera Gel Leave-in Conditioner

Ingredients:

½ cup water

½ cup aloe vera gel

10 drops essential oil (optional)

Add water and aloe vera gel to a small bowl and stir slowly with a spoon. Pour the contents into a spray bottle and shake. Add an essential oil for fragrance and shake again. Use daily or as often as needed to restore softness.

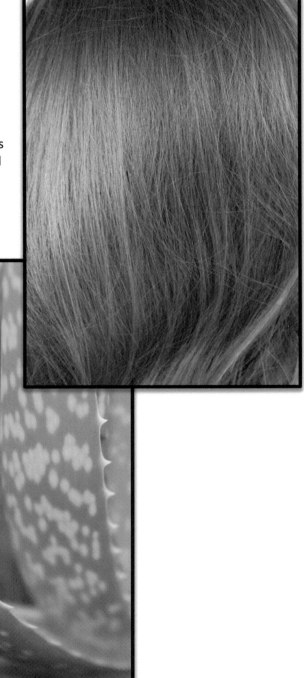

In Mint Condition Leave-In Conditioner

Jojoba Oil and Peppermint Leave-in Conditioner

Ingredients:

2 oz. jojoba oil

4 oz. water

6 drops peppermint essential oil

Combine the ingredients in a bowl and whisk together until well combined. Pour the lotion into a spray bottle and apply the conditioner on your wet locks. Let your tresses dry naturally or use a high-quality hair-dryer. Repeat this ritual at least twice a week for quick results.

Flowery Speeches Leave-In Conditioner

Olive Oil and Safflower Oil Leave-In conditioner

Ingredients:

2 tsp. olive oil

2 oz. Piña Colada Conditioner (see page 22)

2 tsp. safflower oil

1 cup water

Combine all ingredients in a bowl and stir until smooth. Pour the lotion into a spray bottle and apply the conditioner on your wet locks. Let your tresses dry naturally or use a high-quality hair-dryer and repeat this ritual at least twice a week for quick results.

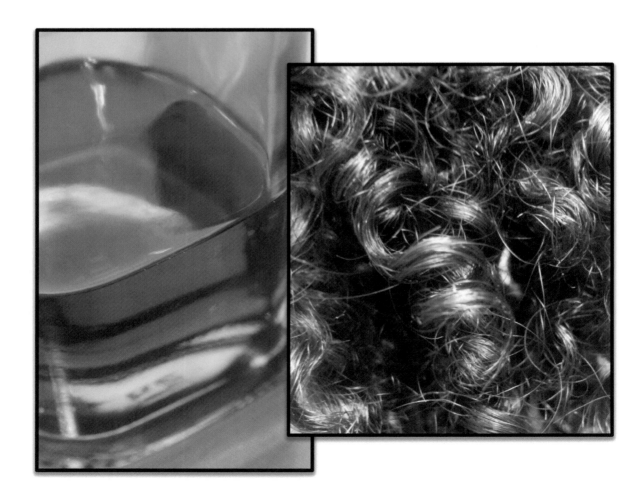

Gummy Bears Conditioner

Slippery Leave-In Conditioner

Ingredients:

1/4 tsp. guar gum

1/4 tsp. xanthan gum

1 tbsp. organic coconut oil

1 cup distilled or purified water

1 tsp. flax oil

3 to 5 drops vanilla essential oil (or the scent of your choice)

Combine the ingredients in a blender. Blend mixture in a blender for 2-5 minutes or until it reaches the consistency you like.

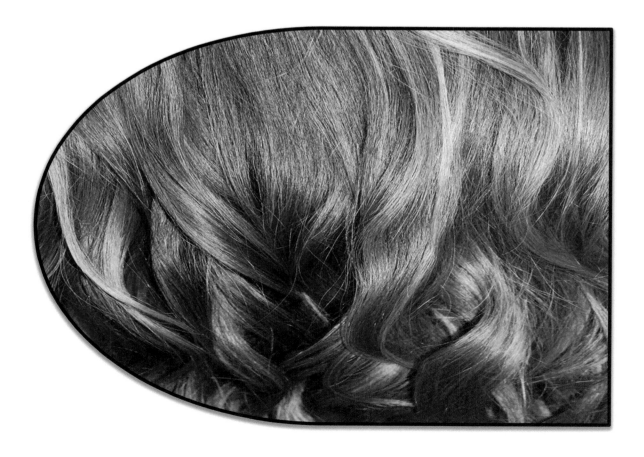

Tasty Treatments
And Rinses

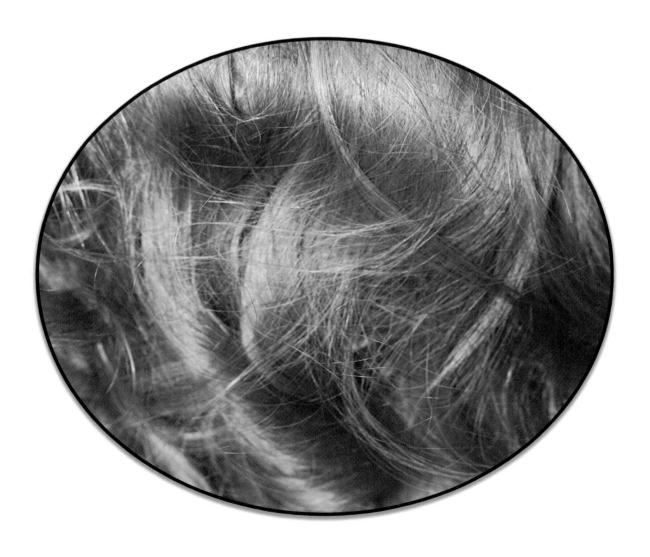

Jolly Jojoba Treatment

Jojoba Hot Oil Treatment

Ingredients:

2 tsp. jojoba oil

1 tsp. organic soybean or sunflower oil

Combine ingredients in a saucepan then warm gently on low heat to lukewarm temperature. Test oil on inside of forearm to ensure oil is not too hot. Massage mixture into hair. Wrap hair in a hot towel or cover with a shower cap or plastic wrap for 15 minutes. Shampoo and rinse out.

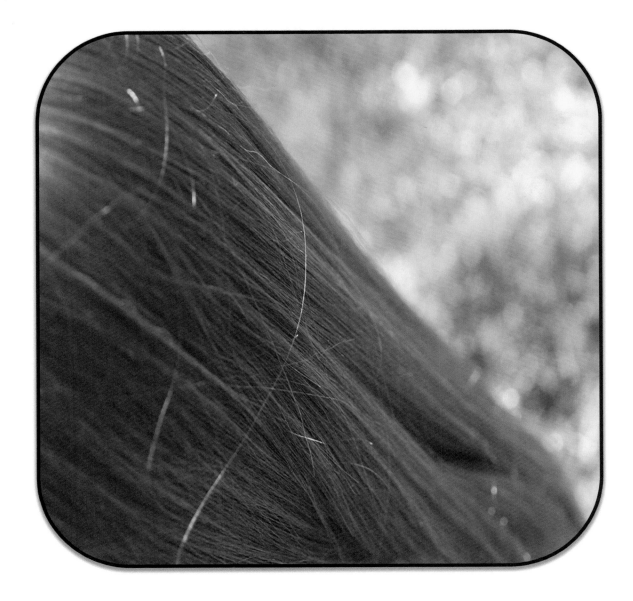

Smells Like Roses Treatment

Rosemary Hot Oil Treatment

Ingredients:

½ cup dried rosemary

½ cup organic soybean or sunflower oil

Combine ingredients in a saucepan and heat until warm. Strain through a fine strainer or cheesecloth. Coat the hair with the oil, working it through to the ends. Wrap hair in plastic wrap followed by a warm towel. Leave oil on for 15 minutes. Shampoo hair until oil is removed.

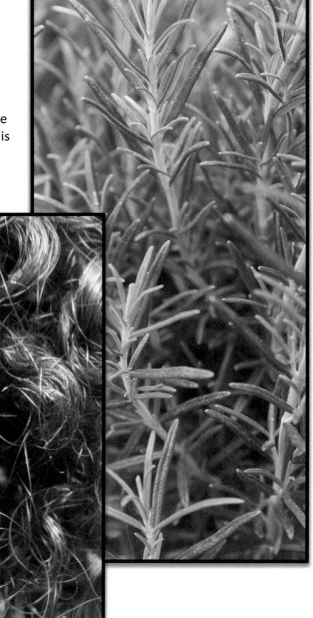

Out of the Sandalwoods Treatment

Hot Oil Treatment For Damaged Hair

Ingredients:

½ cup organic soybean or sunflower oil

8 drops sandalwood essential oil

8 drops lavender essential oil

8 drops geranium essential oil

Mix all ingredients well in a saucepan. Warm mixture to a comfortable temperature then apply it to damp hair. Wrap hair in plastic wrap and apply a hot towel for 20 minutes. Shampoo until oil is removed.

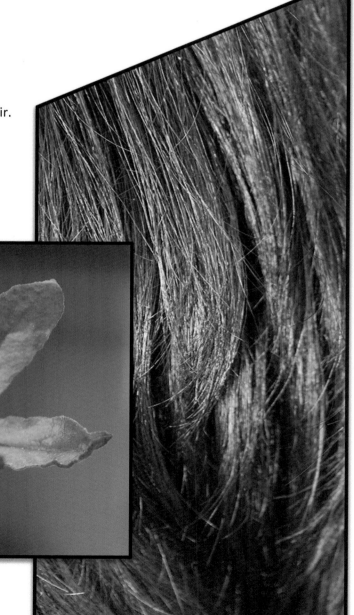

Come Rain or Shine Treatment

Hair Shine Treatment

Ingredients:

2 tsp. fresh rosemary or ½ tsp. dried rosemary

1 cup boiling water

1 tbsp. honey or molasses

1 egg white, lightly beaten

Steep the rosemary in the boiling water for 15 minutes. Pour the water through a strainer and discard the rosemary. Whisk in the honey and egg white until well combined.

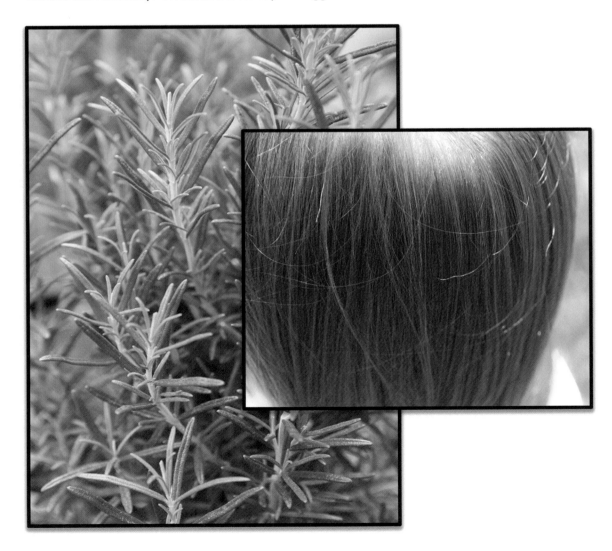

Green with Envy Treatment

Chlorine Treatment

Ingredients:

1 egg, beaten

2 tbsp. olive oil

¼ cup cucumber, peeled and pureed

Combine all ingredients into a medium sized bowl and mix until smooth in texture. Massage into hair from scalp to ends, and then cover with a shower cap. Leave on for 30 minutes at room temperature. Rinse then follow up with Piña Colada Conditioner.

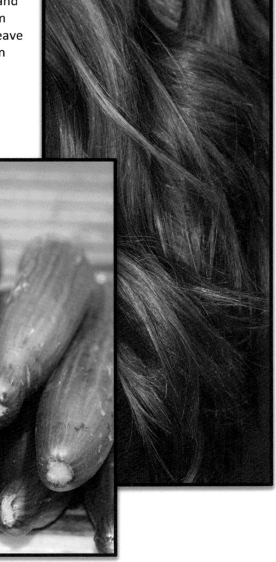

Going to Great Lengths Treatment

Hair Growth Treatment

Ingredients:

3 drops cedarwood essential oil

3 drops lavender essential oil

3 drops lemon essential oil

3 drops rosemary essential oil

3 drops thyme essential oil

1/8 cup grapeseed oil

1/8 cup jojoba oil

Combine all ingredients in a bowl and whisk until well combined. Apply several drops of the mixture to areas of hair loss each night, massaging gently into the scalp for 3-5 minutes. Store oil in an airtight container and keep away from heat and light.

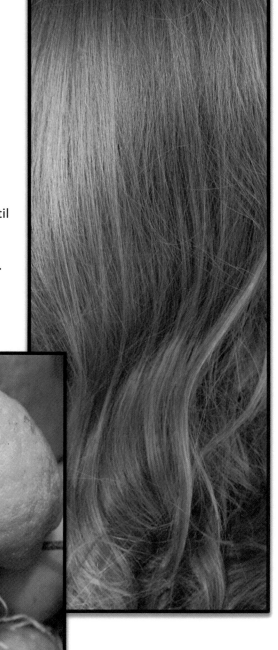

CocoTea Treement

Dandruff Treatment

Ingredients:

¼ cup coconut oil

¼ tsp. tea tree oil

Combine ingredients. Massage into scalp before bed and cover head with a breathable shower cap.

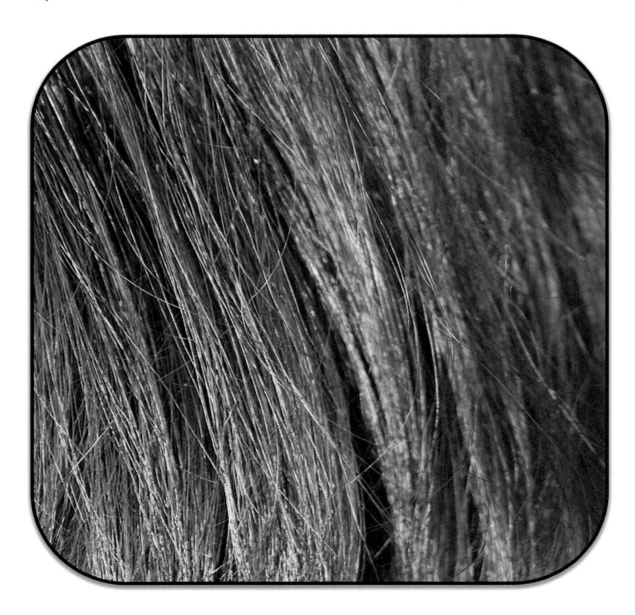

Just Horsing Around Rinse

Bodifying Rinse

Ingredients:

2 ½ tsp. dried horsetail

1 cup water

Steep horsetail in boiling water for 20 minutes. Shampoo hair and rinse thoroughly. Pour rinse through hair and leave in for 10 minutes. Rinse with lukewarm water.

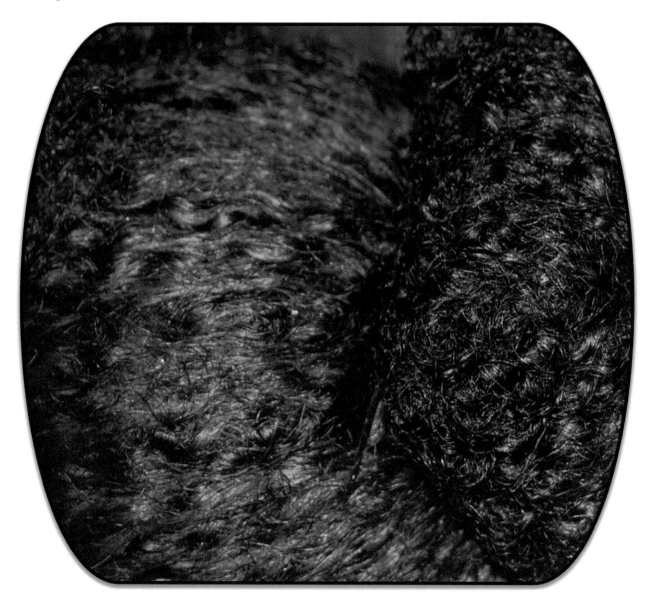

Clean as a Whistle Rinse

Clarifying Rinse

Ingredients:

½ cup apple cider vinegar

1 ½ cups cool water

Mix ingredients in a bottle. Shampoo and rinse hair as usual. Pour vinegar rinse through hair, but do not rinse hair again. (The vinegar scent will dissipate quickly.) The ratio of vinegar to water may be adjusted according to the amount of clarifying needed or frequency of use; add more vinegar if additional clarifying is needed. This rinse will effectively remove product build-up from hair and leave it soft and shiny.

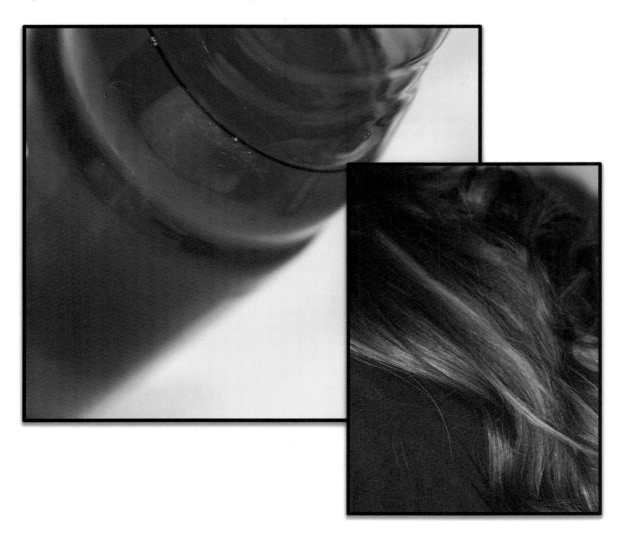

Work Your Soda Off Rinse

Heavy Build-Up Clarifying Rinse

Ingredients:

3 tbsp. baking soda

1 1/2 tsp. creamy honey

1/4 tsp. water

Cider Vinegar Clarifying Hair Rinse

Make one recipe of Clean as a Whistle Rinse. Add the remaining ingredients together to form a paste. Add additional water, a few drops at a time, if the mixture is too thick. Shampoo hair as usual. Apply mixture to hair and leave on for up to five minutes. Rinse hair as usual.

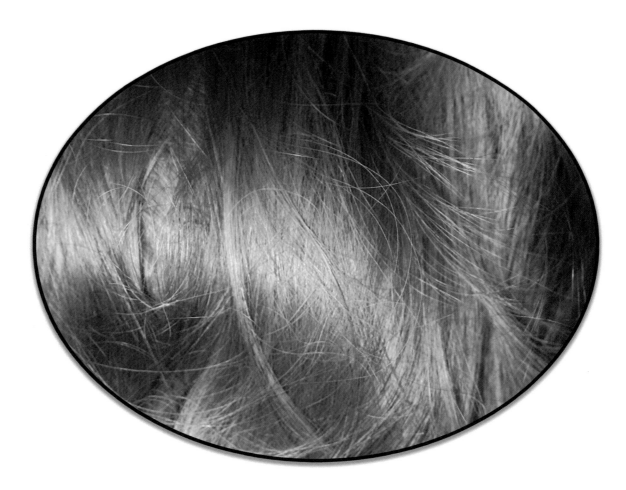

Rinse Before You Leap Rinse

Pre-Poo Oil Rinse

Ingredients:

Olive oil or Jojoba oil

Pour a small amount of oil into the palm of your hand. Rub palms together and gently apply to ends of hair. Let it sit for an hour to allow the oil to penetrate hair strands. Shampoo as usual.

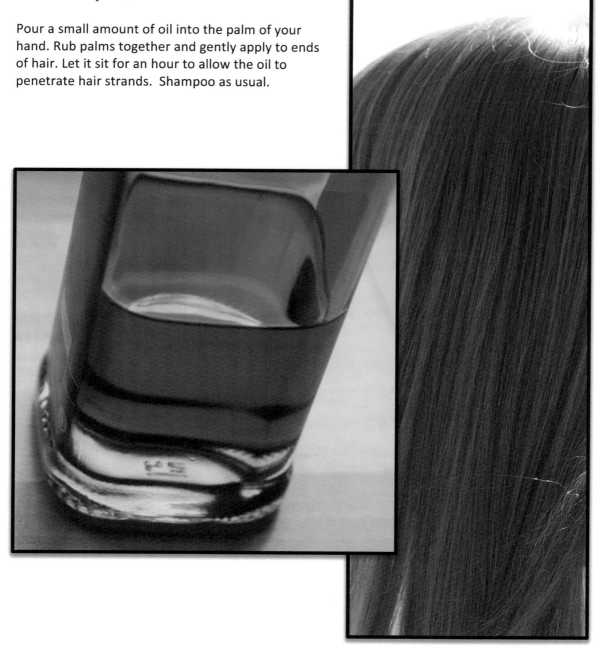

Valuable Vinegar Rinses

Vinegar rinses relieve itchy scalp, dandruff, and dull hair and restore the scalp's natural acid mantle. They are best for normal and oily hair, rather than dry. Use white vinegar for blondes, apple cider vinegar for brunettes, and red wine vinegar for redheads. Leave the rinse on for at least five minutes if you are going to rinse it out. You can, however, leave it on and any smell will dissipate once the hair is dry.

Herb blend:

For blondes: calendula and chamomile

For dark hair: nettle and marshmallow

Vinegar

A few drops essential oil, if desired for fragrance

Distilled water

Fill a quart jar half way with herbs. Cover with vinegar and cap tightly. Place the jar in a warm spot for 2-3 weeks, shaking daily. Strain the vinegar, discarding the herbs and add essential oils. Store in a plastic bottle. Dilute the rinse with distilled water. For oily hair, dilute one part rinse with four parts water. For dry hair, dilute one part rinse with six parts water. After shampooing and rinsing, pour vinegar rinse slowly over hair, massaging it into the scalp. Rinse with water.

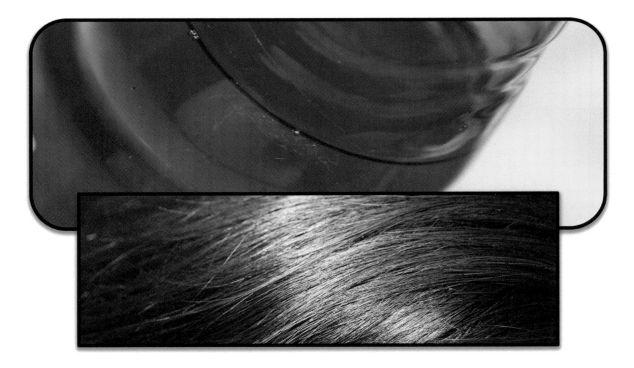

Healthy Herbal Tea Hair Rinse

Anti-Dandruff Herbal Hair Rinse

Ingredients:

1 qt. water

Large handful of rosemary, nettle, thyme, and lavender

2 tbsp. apple cider vinegar or lemon juice, use vinegar if your hair is dry, lemon juice if it is oily.

Bring water to a boil and add the herb mixture. Stir, cover, and steep for 30 minutes. Strain and add either vinegar or lemon juice. After shampooing and conditioning, squeeze out excess water, then pour the liquid over your hair and don't rinse it out.

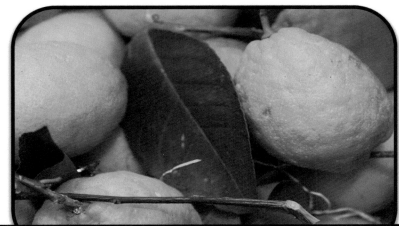

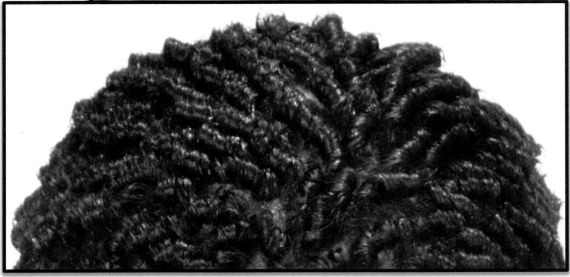

Charming Colors

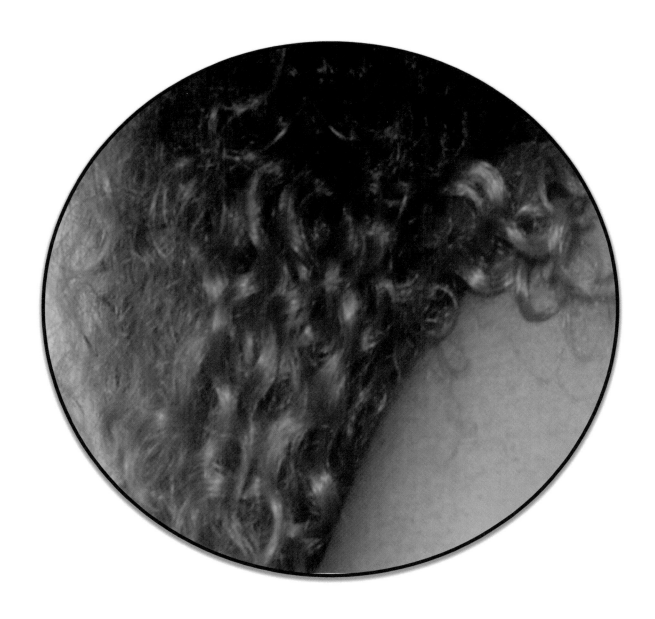

Lightning-Fast Lavender Hair Brightener

Blonde Hair Brightener

Ingredients: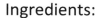

1 cup water

6 organic chamomile tea bags

½ cup plain yogurt

10 drops lavender essential oil

Bring the water to boil and steep tea bags for 15 minutes. Discard tea bags. Combine yogurt, lavender oil and tea, mixing thoroughly. Apply the mixture to dry hair, working through to ends. Cover head with plastic wrap and leave on for 30 minutes. Rinse out and shampoo and condition hair as usual.

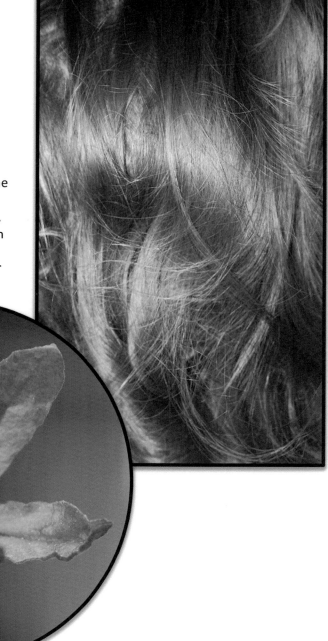

Cup of Joe Hair Dye

Brunette Hair Dye

Ingredients:

2 cups triple strength black coffee

Shampoo hair. Place a large bowl in sink and rinse hair with cooled coffee. Repeat several times, reusing the coffee. Leave final rinse in hair for at least 15 minutes. Rinse with clear water.

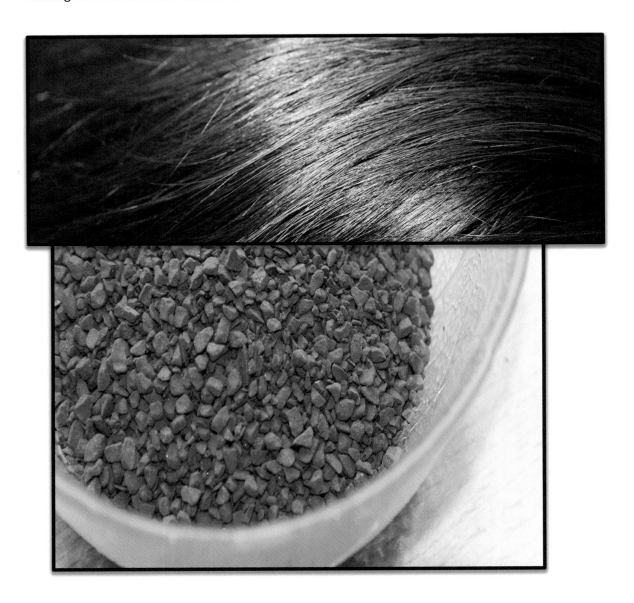

Strawberries for Blondes Hair Dye

Red Color Enhancer

Ingredients:

1/2 cup beet juice

1/2 cup carrot juice

Mix ingredients together and pour over clean, damp hair. Wrap head in plastic and apply hot towel, medium dryer heat, or sit in the sun for one hour. Shampoo and condition hair.

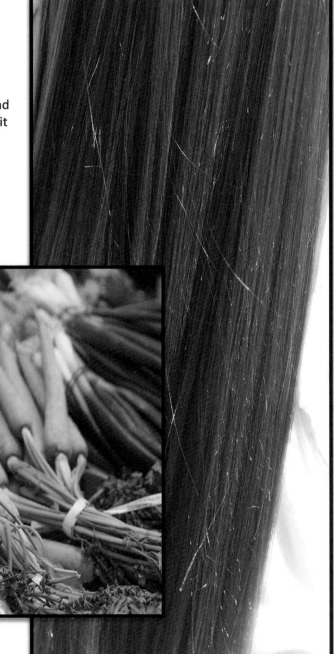

Hearty Henna Hair Dye

Conditioning Hair Color

Ingredients:

3.5 oz. henna in powder form

Piña Colada Conditioner (see page 22)

Mix henna using half the water as directed on the package. Add conditioner to the mixture until your desired consistency is reached. Apply to hair, working through hair thoroughly. Leave on hair following directions on henna package. Rinse henna from hair and follow with shampoo. May be used with colorless henna to increase volume of fine hair without adding color.

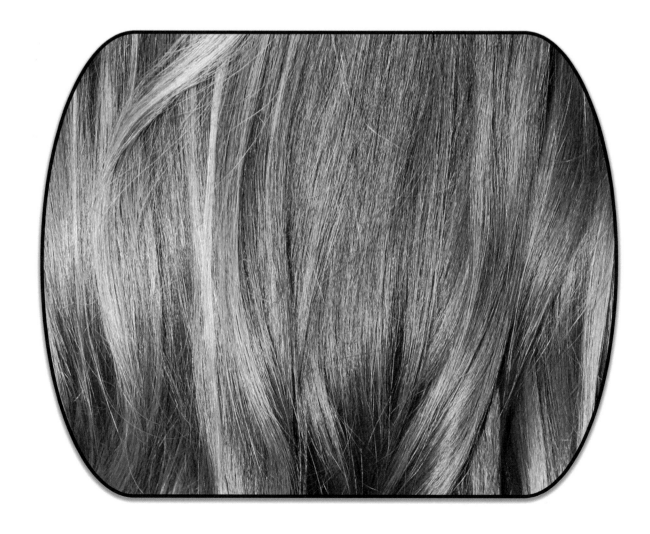

Sage Advice Natural Restorer

Natural Restorer For Gray Hair

Ingredients:

½ cup dried sage

½ cup dried rosemary

2 cups water

Simmer rosemary and sage in water for 30 minutes then steep for several hours. Apply to gray hair and allow to dry, then shampoo and condition hair. Repeat weekly until desired shade is reached, then once a month for maintenance.

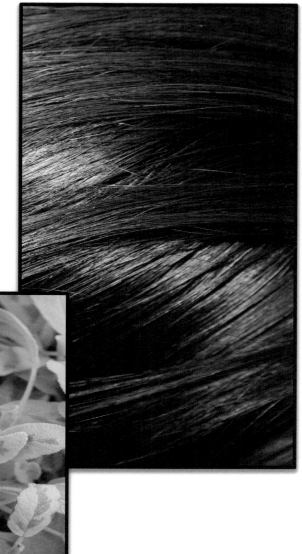

Spicy Cinnamon Bears Temporary Color

Cinnamon Brown

Ingredients:

1 tbsp. cinnamon powder

1 tsp. cocoa power

1 tsp. nutmeg powder

2 tsp. cornstarch

15 drops lavender or rosemary essential oil

1 empty makeup compact

1 compact sponge

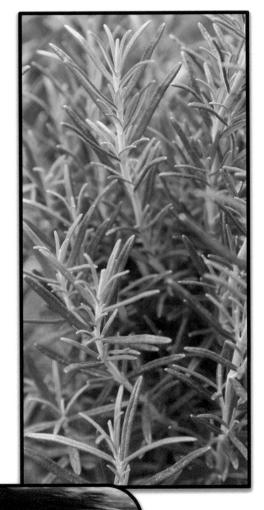

Combine powders into a small bowl and mix. Add more cocoa, nutmeg and/or cinnamon to reach your desired hue. Once you have reached the desired color, press powder into a compact and seal with 15 drops of essential oil. Close the compact and let it sit for 24 hours to allow for the powder to set. When ready to use on dry styled hair, grab strands of hair and add highlights by opening the compact and sliding the open compact down the strand of the hair to release the color. Grab bigger chunks of hair for a more all over colored look.

Honey Butter Temporary Color

Honey Blonde

Ingredients:

1 tbsp. cinnamon powder

2 tsp. turmeric

2 tsp. cornstarch

15 drops lavender or rosemary essential oil

1 empty makeup compact

1 compact sponge

Combine powders into a small bowl and mix. Add more turmeric or cinnamon to reach your desired hue. Once you have reached the desired color, press powder into a compact and seal with 15 drops of essential oil. Close the compact and let it sit for 24 hours to allow for the powder to set. When ready to use on dry styled hair, grab strands of hair and add highlights by opening the compact and sliding the open compact down the strand of the hair to release the color. Grab bigger chunks of hair for a more all over colored look.

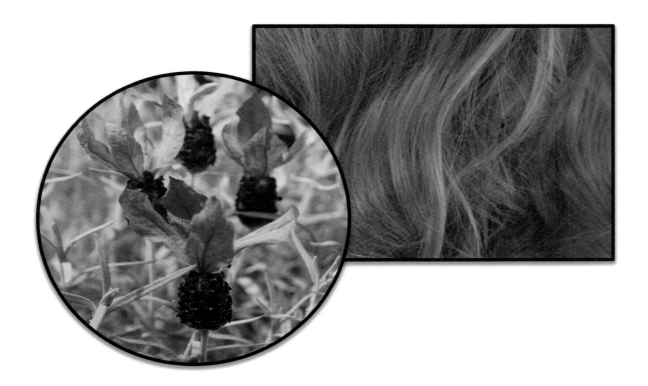

Succulent Styling Products

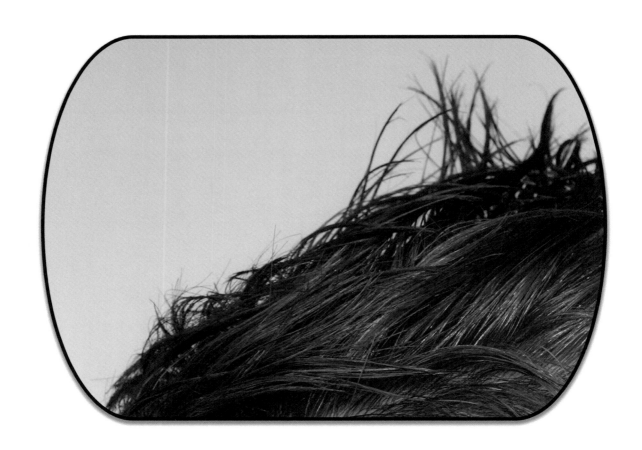

Ain't It Amazing Aloe Detangler

Aloe Detangler

Ingredients:

1 cup distilled water

2 tbsp. aloe vera gel

4 drops vegetable glycerin

Mix all ingredients together and pour into an old shampoo bottle and shake until everything is well blended. A spray bottle works well too. Squeeze or spray it onto your hands and then work the detangler through the hair with your fingers. Detangle as normal; do not rinse.

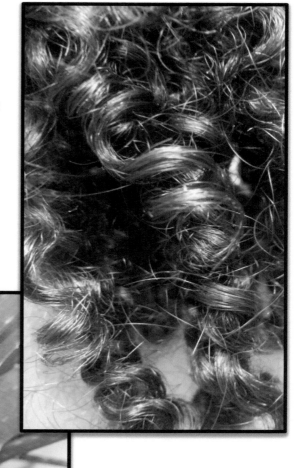

Grab Me Some Grapefruit Detangler

Basic Hair Detangler

Ingredients:

1 tsp. aloe vera gel

½ tsp. grapefruit seed extract

2 drops grapefruit essential oil

2 drops glycerin

1 cup purified water

Mix all ingredients together and pour into an old shampoo bottle and shake until everything is well blended. A spray bottle works well too. Squeeze or spray the detangler onto your hands and work it through the hair with your fingers. Detangle as normal; do not rinse.

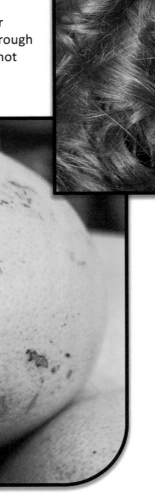

Flax Them Muscles Gel

Flax Seed Gel

Ingredients:

2 tbsp. whole flax seeds

1 cup water

Aloe vera gel (optional)

Essential oil (optional, for fragrance)

Boil water then pour in the flax seeds. Stirring constantly, allow the flax seeds to boil in the water until a gel consistency starts to occur, boiling about 5 minutes. DO NOT OVER COOK. Strain the gel from the flax seeds using a fine-mesh sieve. Place in a squeeze or pump bottle, and add aloe vera gel to flax seed gel. Add up to 4 drops of your favorite essential oil. Shake well. Use as you would any hair gel.

*For extra softness with hold, add ½ tbsp. aloe vera gel per 2 tbsp. flax seed gel.
**For thicker gel, use 3 tbsp. whole flax seeds to 1 cup water ratio.
***You must refrigerate the gel to preserve and reuse.

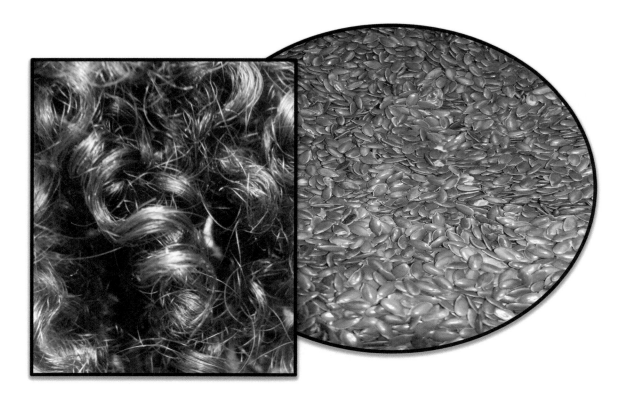

All-Nighter Agar Agar Gel

Agar Agar Hair Gel

Ingredients:

½ cup Agar Agar (concentration of choice)

¼ cup aloe vera gel

10 drops essential oil (optional, for fragrance)

Prepare ½ cup Agar Agar as instructed on package, usually by simmering and stirring. When all the agar flakes are dissolved, remove from heat and whisk in aloe vera and essential oil. Pour mixture into an airtight container and refrigerate at least 6 hours.

*For a "normal hold" hair gel, use the Agar Agar at the concentration listed on the package. For an even tougher product, you can mix up a batch at 150% or 200% concentration.

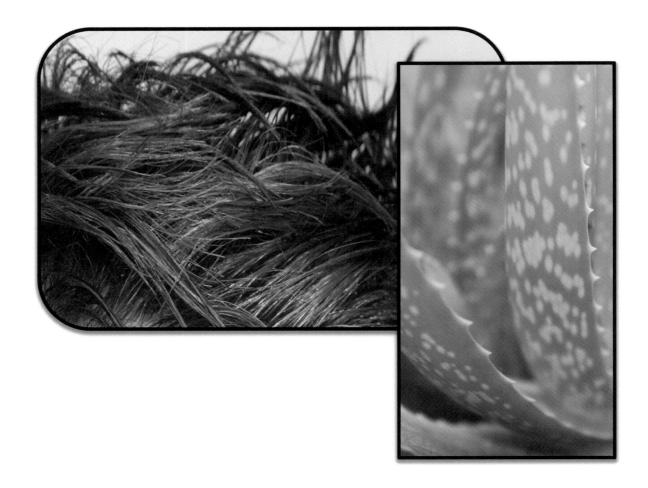

Oh My Goodness Gracious Gel

Gelatin Hair Gel

Ingredients:

½ tsp. unflavored gelatin

1 cup warm water

Dissolve gelatin in water. Keep refrigerated and use as you would any hair gel.
*For a thicker hair gel, use 1 tsp. gelatin.

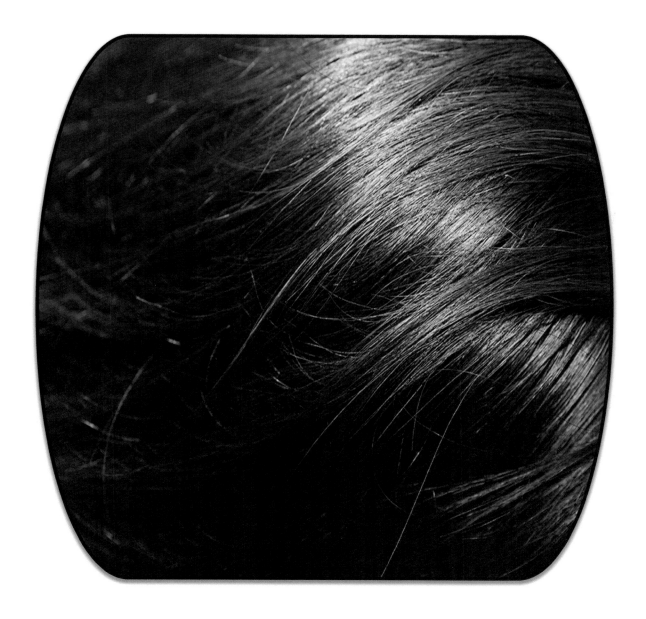

Get a Fix On It Gel

Aloe Gel For Edge Control

Ingredients:

½ cup aloe vera gel

3 tbsp. jojoba oil

3 tbsp. vegetable glycerin

¼ tsp. xanthum gum

Add all ingredients to a mixing bowl and mix using a hand mixer on low setting. The xanthum gum will add thickness to the recipe; adjust how much you use to get the consistency you want. Thickening the consistency of the gel makes it easier to control the application and get the aloe exactly to the areas needed. The added glycerin also helps seal in the other elements.

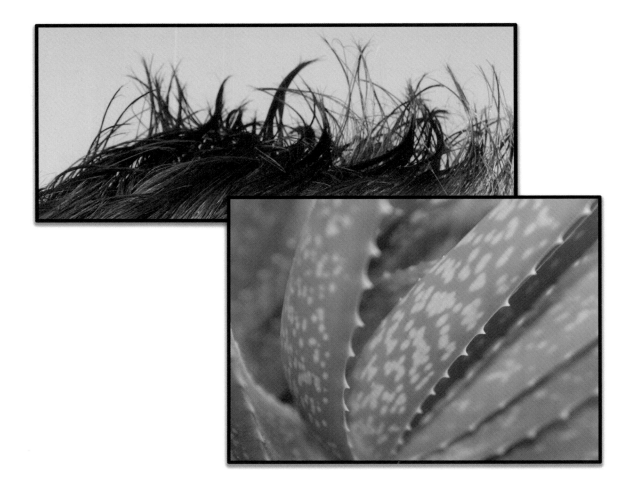

Hair Raisin' Spritz

Aloe Hair Spritz

Ingredients:

½ cup aloe vera gel

½ cup distilled water

1-2 tbsp. Flowery Speeches Leave-In Conditioner (see page

41)

Add all ingredients to a spray bottle and shake to mix. It takes a few minutes for the aloe and conditioner to mix completely. Ensure the mixture is completely blended before using.

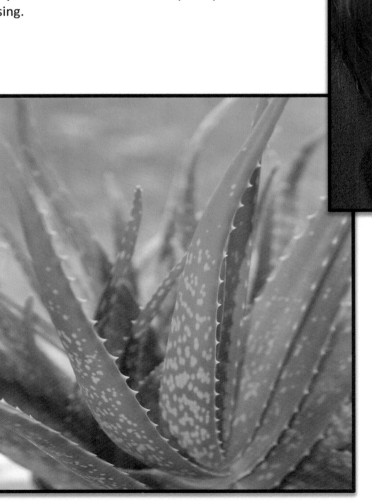

Smooth Operator Serum

Simple Smoothing Serum

Ingredients:

Vitamin E Oil

Apply a small dollop of pure vitamin E oil to the center of your palm. Rub your hands together, and then run both palms over your hair, starting at the roots and moving down. For split or dry ends, apply a bit more vitamin E directly to the tips of your hair as well.

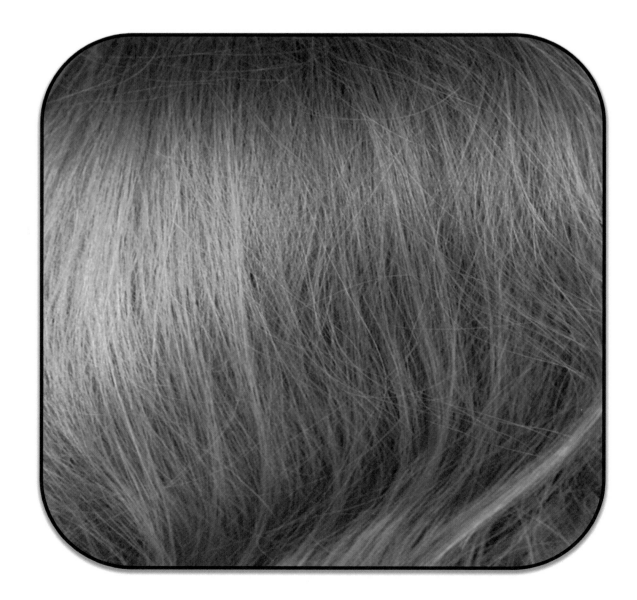

Straight as a Pin Serum

Hair Serum For Sleek, Straight Hair

Ingredients:

½ cup distilled water

½ cup aloe vera gel

2 tsp. grapeseed oil

4 drops essential oil (optional, for fragrance)

Add ingredients to blender and blend until well combined. Apply to damp hair, focusing on the ends, before blow drying.

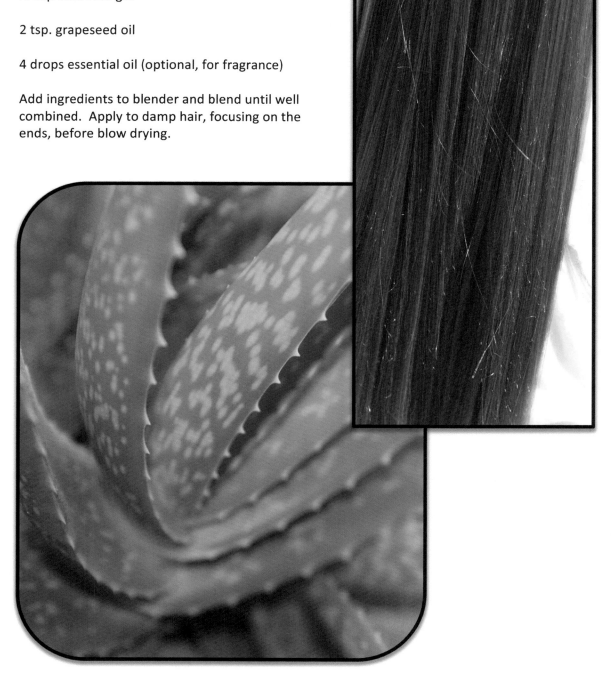

Butter Up Your Hair

Natural Hair Grease

Ingredients:

2 oz. lanolin oil

1 oz. raw, unrefined shea butter

1 ½ tsp. extra virgin olive oil

½ tsp. apple pie spice (optional, for fragrance)

Heat and melt the shea butter using a double boiler or improvised double boiler method. Stir in remaining ingredients then pour the mixture into container and allow it to cool. Add any desired fragrance when mixture is cool and begins to thicken and solidify.

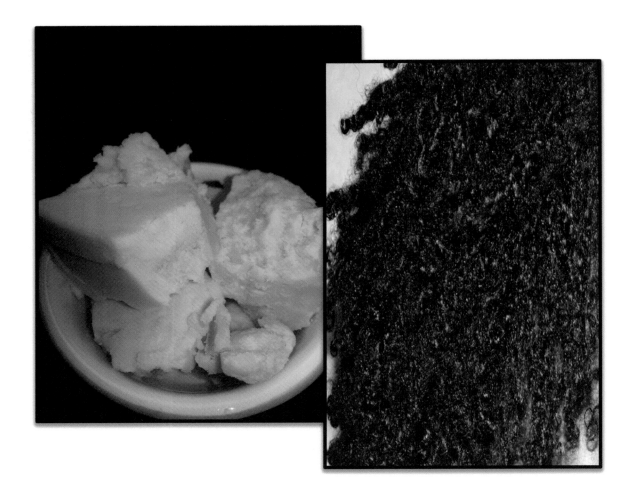

Castor a Spell on Your Curls

Curling and Twisting Cream

Ingredients:

1 tbsp. castor oil

¼ cup shea butter

1 ¼ cup Flax Them Muscles Gel

Whisk the shea butter with the castor oil using a hand mixer. Add the gel to the mixture and mix until well combined. Use to define curls or apply before twisting for a defined twist-out or before braiding for hold.

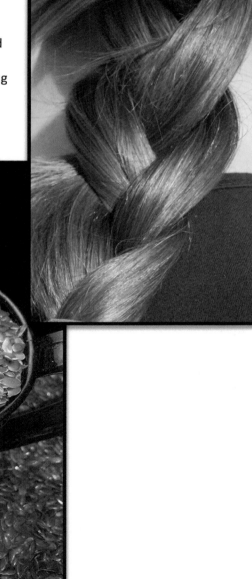

Helpful
Hints

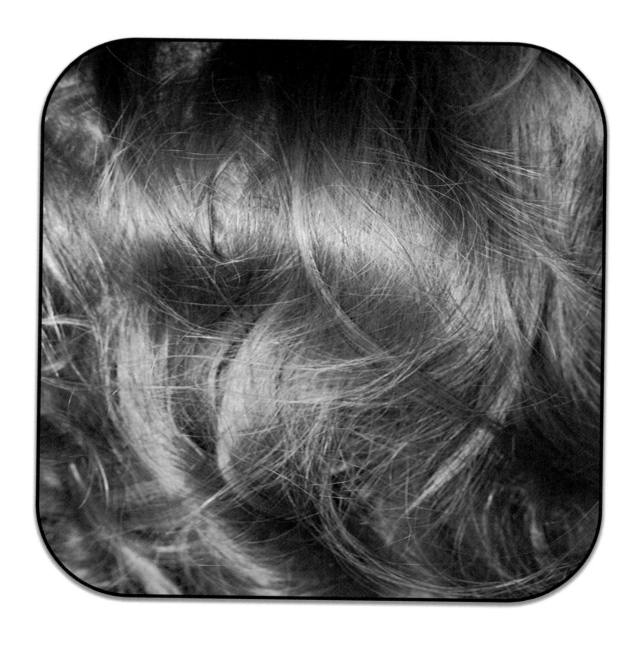

General Hair Information and Tips

❀ Hair is made up of protein (95-97% protein and 3% water). Be sure you are getting enough of it. Other hair essentials include: biotin (eggs, organ meats, dried fruit, molasses), iron, iodine, B12, and Omega 3s.

❀ Teas to improve hair health include: alfalfa, burdock root, *ho shou wu*, horsetail, nettle, and oat straw.

❀ Seaweed is said to keep hair healthy and dark.

❀ Rinsing hair with cold water will flatten hair and make it better able to reflect light.

❀ Scalp massages can prevent hair loss, stimulate sebaceous glands, and increase circulation. Add a few drops of rosemary essential oil to fingertips to enhance a massage.

❀ Brushing hair distributes hair oils. Natural bristles are best because they absorb and distribute the oils and trap dirt and dust.

❀ Minimize blow dryers, hot rollers, curling irons, and chlorinated swimming pools. When using a blow dryer hold it at least 6 inches away from the hair and use a low heat setting.

❀ Reduce stress in your life, which can cause hair loss and lackluster hair. Yoga, meditation, massage, and a cup of calming tea are wonderful ways to combat stress.

❀ Get your hair trimmed every eight weeks to remove frizzy, split, or frayed ends.

❀ Wear a hat to protect your hair from sunlight, which can be drying or color changing (especially for color treated hair).

Beneficial Hair Product Ingredients

❀ Avocado provides essential vitamins and minerals that are essential for healthy hair. It contains B vitamins, beta-carotene, copper, vitamin E, vitamin C, and essential fatty acids, all of which will strengthen and fortify hair.

❀ A ripe banana is included in the recipe to help soften hair and protect its natural elasticity. Bananas are rich in potassium, natural oils, carbohydrates and vitamins, which will help not only bring out the shine but also control dandruff and promote hair growth.

❀ Coconut milk also helps control dandruff and promotes hair growth and the protein and other nutrients soften hair.

❀ Olive oil moisturizes dry, damaged hair and is one of the best sources of omega-9 fatty acids.

❀ Egg yolks also have naturally occurring fatty acts and are naturally rich in vitamin A, D, E and B vitamins, which are all beneficial for improving hair's appearance.

❀ For people with excessive oily hair, egg whites can be applied to the roots. Egg whites are full of bacteria-eating enzymes that will help get rid of unnecessary dirt and oils.

❀ Apple cider vinegar kills germs and helps to remove any excess buildup of previous shampoos or conditioners. This tends to make the hair lighter, shinier and easier to manage.

❀ Lemon juice adds an extra fight against dandruff and also strengthens hair roots.

❀ Beer contains proteins that repair hair while the sugars in the beer make hair shiny by tightening the hair cuticles.

❀ A drop or two of the lavender essential oil is very relaxing and calming to the body and mind and adds that luxurious touch to this pampering hair care treatment.

❀ Mayonnaise is a well-known hair revitalizer. Rub mayonnaise into wet hair after shampooing, and let it set for 15-20 minutes with a shower cap or plastic bag. Rinse out with warm water. This will condition your hair leaving it stronger, healthier and full of moisture.

❀ Combining coconut milk & lemon juice works wonders for frizzy hair. Mix a cup of coconut milk with a tablespoon of lemon juice then warm the mixture to a lukewarm temperature. Rub this mixture into your hair and scalp, leave on for 20 minutes and rinse with warm water. This treatment can be used on wet or dry hair as a pre-shampoo or post-shampoo conditioner.

❀ Eggs have a high sulfur content, which can help you grow your hair longer and stronger. For a deep conditioner, beat two eggs and whisk in a tablespoon of honey. Use the mixture on damp or wet hair. Rub the egg into your hair and scalp, and cover with a shower cap. Let it set for 20 minutes and rinse. It gives gloss to your hair and nice volume.

❀ Baking soda absorbs grease, dirt and excess oil in hair.

❀ Grapeseed oil has a very high smoking point (420º F), so it makes it a good protectant against the heat of blow-drying.

❀ Grapefruit seed extract is a natural preservative that protects the shampoo from bacteria growth.

About the Author

Dezarae Henderson, MBA, developed a passion for styling hair at the age of twelve.   A self proclaimed former "Product Junkie", she searched for and purchased hair products claiming to tame her natural hair. After years of chemically processing her hair to achieve certain styles and not achieving ideal outcomes, she decided to take matters into her own hands and make natural hair products. This gave her the opportunity to ensure the ingredients were 100% natural and allowed her to customize recipes to suit her hair needs. Once she took a more natural approach to caring for her hair, Dezarae has grown healthy hair ever since.   As a result of numerous requests for hair consultations and advice, Dezarae decided to share these recipes with all of the women searching for answers to managing healthy natural hair. Now, every woman has a little Kitchen Beautician inside of them. This cookbook is just for you!

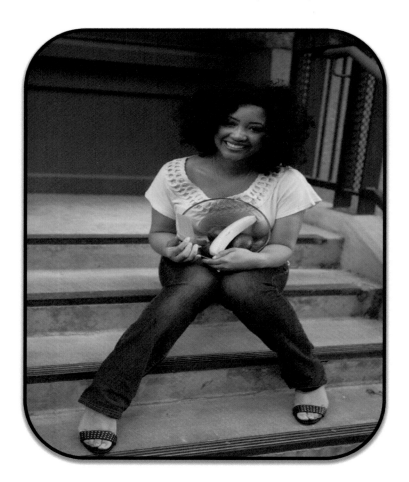